Also by Tricia Hersey

Rest Is Resistance: A Manifesto

We will Rest!

The Art of Escape

Tricia Hersey

Art by George McCalman

Little, Brown Spark

New York Boston London

To Saheim the Dream and other dreamers like Miss Tubman. Follow the light.

Harriet was now left alone...She turned her face toward the north, and fixing her eyes on the guiding star, and committing her way unto the Lord, she started again upon her long, lonely journey... "For," said she, "I had reasoned dis out in my mind; there was one of two things I had a *right* to, liberty, or death."

—from *Harriet, the Moses of Her People*

by SARAH H. BRADFORD

If the enslaved could believe, I know I can.

—NIKKI GIOVANNI

WE WILL REST

Q

HOW DO YOU FIND
REST
IN A CAPITALIST, WHITE SUPREMACIST, PATRIARCHAL, ABLEIST SYSTEM?

WE WILL REST

A

YOU TAP INTO YOUR TRICKSTER ENERGY. YOU BECOME AN ESCAPE ARTIST.

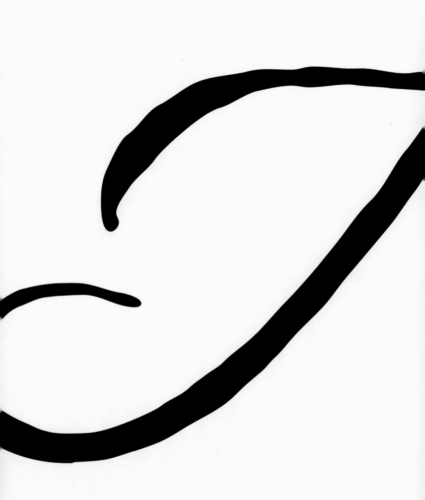

WE WILL REST

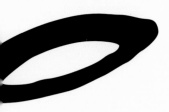

This book is a sacred object.

You are a sacred object.

This book is a manual on care.

You are an escape artist.

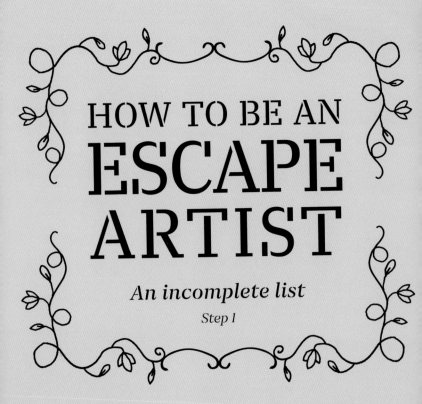

HOW TO BE AN
ESCAPE
ARTIST

An incomplete list

Step 1

WE WILL REST

The first step for morphing into an escape artist is belief. You must believe you have the power to refuse. You must believe you have been gifted with everything necessary. You must be a trickster. No matter what, you must not show fear. We are abundant. I have heard from many that it's been difficult to rest because you don't know how. Give thanks for the "not knowing." Isn't it exciting to be able to develop, discover, and experiment with your own liberation?

I am the trickster.

The one who got away.

The one who always knew.

The one able to transmute grief to rest.

I am the trickster.

The one who refused.

The one leaping from the tops of mountains

Into a bed of feather pillows.

I am the trickster.

Assigned as the debt collector

By my Ancestors.

Resting to reclaim the DreamSpace stolen.

Pay up!

I am the trickster.

The one who squinted her eyes.

Cocked her head.

Recognized the lies.

Peeped the scam.

YOU ARE HERE. Thank you for living. Thank you for **RESISTING.** Thank you for caring for each other. Thank you, **DIVINE.** Thank you for **ABUN-DANCE.** Thank you for **RESTING.** For silence, for abolition, for sleep, for Sabbath. For **DAYDREAMING.** For **IMAGINATION WORK.** For **ANCES-TORS' WORK.** For subversion. For **ESCAPE.** For thriving in a culture focused on destruction. For **FREE-DOM-DREAMING.** For embodiment. For **DIS-TURBING** the idea that we are powerless. Thank you for your **MARRONAGE.** Thank you for your **REST.** For your love practices. For **TRANSFORMATION.** For slowing down. For remixing oppression to **LIBERA-TION.** The time to Rest is **NOW.**

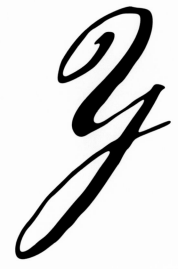

You are Divine.

Let that soak in for three minutes.

I hold back spring while

you soak.

YOU ARE A MIRACLE IN LIGHT.

NO EDITS
NECESSARY
NOT NEEDING TO BE FIXED.

Y ou are archive

Protected document

WE WILL REST

All is well

Will you rest?

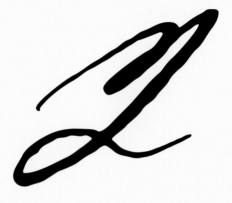

I'm writing this book so you will know you are not unreasonable. That you are not imagining things. That your body is tired, and your mind and spirit feel numb because the systems want it that way. They have worn you down into a pulp. There is life after death. There is spiritual resurrection.

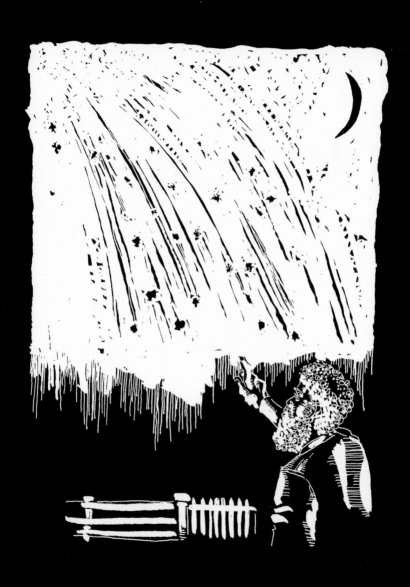

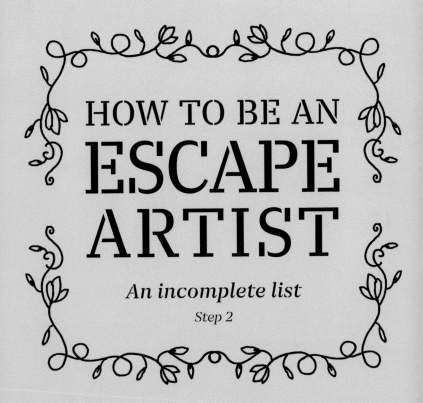

HOW TO BE AN ESCAPE ARTIST

An incomplete list

Step 2

WE WILL REST

Develop clear boundaries that feel like fresh clay. Flexible, strong, and soothing to your body. Develop the ability to ignore anyone and anything that stands in the way of your goal of liberation. Every system in the culture doesn't see your divinity. They were not created to connect. They were not created to have vision. They were created for you to internalize the lies about labor in a capitalist culture. Stay clear. Stay connected.

Have you ever noticed

when you ask for rest

the body becomes a holy trumpet?

The walls come tumbling down.

I wish we didn't need
AN ESCAPE MANUAL.
I wish we didn't need
AN ESCAPE PLAN.
I wish we didn't need
TO STEAL AWAY AND SNATCH REST.
I wish we didn't have
TO DISRUPT THE LIES OF GRIND CULTURE.
I wish we didn't need
TO OVERWORK TO EAT.
I wish we didn't feel
LIKE OUR BODIES BELONG TO CAPITALISM.
I wish we didn't have
TO LOOK OUTSIDE OURSELVES.
I wish we didn't need
TO RECLAIM OUR PRECIOUS, FRAGILE, AND DIVINE BODIES.
I wish we didn't need
TO RESIST.

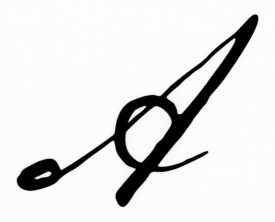

Are you also exhausted? Are you waiting for permission to slow down? Are you waiting to save up enough money and time off from work to fly away to an expensive retreat in another land? Are you waiting for the powers that be to create policies that are drenched with care and room for you to get off the grind? Are you feeling guilt and shame when you rest? Are you hoping for deliverance from pushing through at all costs? Are you waiting for permission?

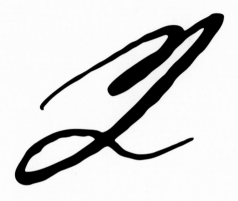

If you are waiting for permission, listen closely: You are enough right now and you must rest not to gain more power or to produce more but because it is your Divine right to rest. Go lay down or close your eyes and daydream right after reading this.

YOU HAVE TIME. THERE IS ALWAYS TIME. THERE IS NO URGENCY.

WE WILL REST

Framing rest as:

Something beautiful.

Something worthy.

Something human.

Something holy.

Something honorable.

Something healing.

Something radical.

Something transformative.

Something attainable.

Something close.

Something powerful.

ODE T
ANCE

WE WILL REST

O MY

TORS

Cotton-picking machines.

My Ancestors.

In the South.

You human machines.

Worked for free.

Enslaved.

Commodified.

DreamSpace theft.

I will never forget.

I will nap for you.

Someone must rest for you.

We will be resurrected there.

This is reparations.

This is rebellion.

Let them come.

Let them rest now.

They are here now.

They are napping with us.

For the millions of enslaved Africans

Laboring on cotton plantations for centuries.

Backbreaking, soul-killing work.

Sharecropping on land that you should have owned.

Robbery.

Building this land.

You are welcomed.

To rest.

BEWARE!

WE WILL REST

Our rest memories are creating the future.

Our memories are creating the future.

Rest is creating our future.

To be an outlier from grind culture requires flexibility, grace, and a trickster energy.

The systems will not offer you rest.

The systems will not make space for your care.

The systems will not see the brilliance of your divinity.

The systems worship capitalism.

May the violent energy cease.

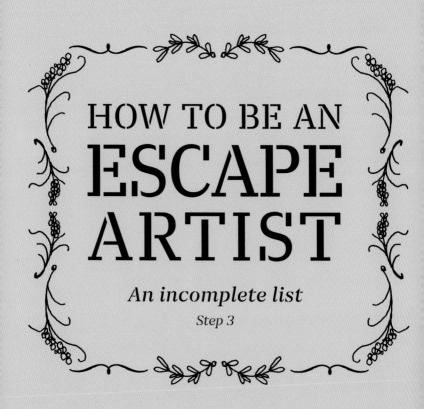

HOW TO BE AN ESCAPE ARTIST

An incomplete list

Step 3

WE WILL REST

Create community. Build community. Be community.
Community care can seem impossible when you are
exhausted. It is possible. Community is anywhere two or
more are gathered. Two is still community. Don't rush
to quantity as the marker of deep community and care.
Don't rush to do anything alone. To be an escape artist
is to be in the collective. Supported in rest, care, and
love. Demand the collective as a source of inspiration
and change. Real change comes from the people.

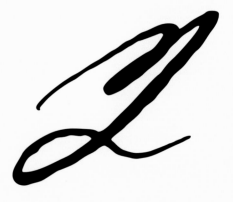

I have claimed myself as an escape artist. My early days experimenting with rest came quickly as the whispering yell of my body lit a path. This is a meditation on how I escaped grind culture. How I built a home by laying down and slowing down and daydreaming in my own community and in my own heart. My deliverance out of grind culture is a spark for my soul.

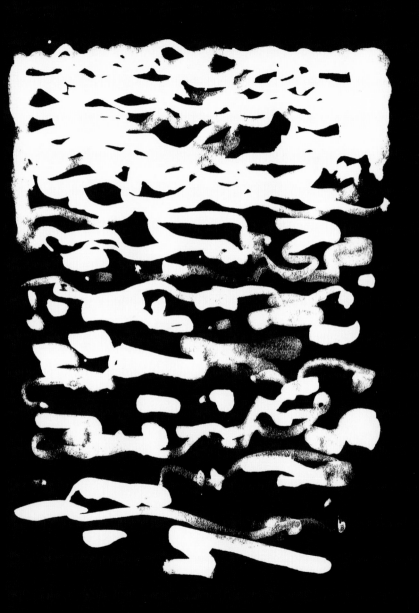

AN ESCAPE PRACTICE

WE WILL REST

Rub your hands together and create energy and heat. Then rub this energy all over your body slowly. Now lay down for three minutes as you breathe deeply. Then rub your hands together more, then breathe and rub this heat over your face slowly. Breathe as deep as you can from your belly. Exhale. You can breathe through anything. Now sit with a partner and ask consent for touch. Now let them put their hands on your back as you breathe. Let them feel your alive-ness.

There is a dialogue that happens when you focus on your breathing and when you focus on being alive. This is the art of escape: to heal, to rest, to desire care.

Wonder

Ain't

to Sa

WE WILL REST

Woman Coming e Us!

We are drowning as

capitalism seeks to automate us

And end us if we can't keep up like robots

Real slow brainwashing-type emergency

I'm amazed

At the survival

I wanna save one million

Of mine

Sorry, but I'm selfish

If you poor and not rich

If you working but still broke

If you tired but still going

Don't wait on Wonder Woman

Or recognition

May never come

Instead become real good at dog-paddling

Learn how to bandage up a wound

That really needs stitches

WE WILL REST

Learn to rest even when you are called lazy
Learn how to slow down even when
the monster of guilt appears

Learn to morph into an escape artist
Learn to refuse the lies of grind culture

We can remix the oppression
Dress up in superhero armor
Pillows, dreams, refusal, and soft blankets
guide our missions

You don't know about survival until you in it
You don't know thriving is possible until you demand it

Wonder Woman ain't coming to save us
She would drown in much exhaustion
Can you blame her?

We must put ourselves in a rest-and-care trance
Walk the streets and swaddle the Shorties up in blankets
Build community centers with our bare hands
Lay down and nap and plot deep plans in our dreams

About Revival

Renewal

Revolution

Resistance

Rest

This is deep

We drowning-type deep

Lungs filling with salt water deep

Deep like flesh and blood on your hands and face

Warrior-like deep

Deeper than all oceans combined

Learning the truth

Now you gotta change all your thinking

Deep

No wreckage and bones in water to hang on for dear life

We haven't checked ourselves

So we are seriously wrecking ourselves

Have you noticed no one is coming?

Wonder Woman ain't coming to save us

We must pop lock and transform into our own superheroes

We must lay down and dream our own selves free

Super South Side Saver

Poor People Lover

Black Freedom Captain

Minister of Dream Revival Services

Rest and Care Queen

Lover of Self-Actualization

Prophetess of Joy

Are you listening?

I'm screaming

Save Ourselves!

We should be a lil' more outraged

Should be resting and daydreaming more

Should proclaim we will never, ever donate our bodies

Merge Manifestos

Create long- and short-term projects

I'm passing out pillows, blankets, and three-ring binders

Filling them with solutions

Carry it around like your new bible

So serious

So wake up

To go lay down

No more shame

No more guilt

No more waiting

No more asking

Rest Now!

Wonder Woman ain't coming to save us

No angel in saint's clothing either

No man on white horse will come flying

No system able to see your divinity

I don't blame individuals

I'm blaming the systems

Real change is when we do it ourselves

An everlasting authentic change

WE WILL REST

Put soapboxes on street corners and it changes

Ask community to not go hard

Get settled

Get pissed

Get clear

Get dreaming

One-track minded

Solve problems

Understand solutions

And rest

I'm on autopilot

Others don't concern me

Survival of the fittest

You are the Wonder

We are the Wonder

We now have the power and tools

The Lasso of Truth

The Golden Escape Plan

The Downloads

The DreamSpace

The Motivation

The Time

The Focus

Flip the script

Wonder Woman ain't coming

We already here!

We Will Rest!

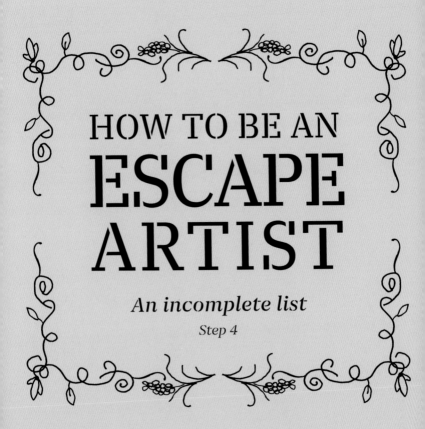

HOW TO BE AN ESCAPE ARTIST

An incomplete list

Step 4

Study the art of improvisation. You will need it for your escape artist life. There are no quick steps or cookie-cutter lies to liberation. You do what you must in the moment and right now. You tap deeply into your inner knowing. You view rest not as an afterthought and instead as the foundation and North Star. Follow the stars. Follow the light. You boldly step into your role as the leader. You carry your escape plan in your pocket. You carry your escape plan in your heart.

SYMBOLS
TO DRAW
IN THE SKY

WE WILL REST

Deliverance

Out of bondage

Magician

Reinvention

Resurrection from death of exhaustion

Spectacle

Creativity

Subversive

Rest as a Freedom Practice

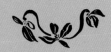

AN ESCAPE PRACTICE

WE WILL REST

Wake up every day and imagine the alternative to grinding and overworking. What would happen if you woke up from a nap and capitalism as we know it was gone? What would future-casting yourself as if you have already escaped feel like? Be the watcher. Ask questions and stand in your dignity. Tell your side of the story before they can taint it.

THE ESCAPE PLAN
BEGINS

The couch as refuge

The dark brown couch sat very low to the wooden floor in our small living room. It became an altar for my rest experiments. A knowing that I no longer could exist in the unsustainable pace of a life controlled by capitalism. Every day, I would lay flat on the couch no matter what time it was. Each day consisted of making sure my son was off to elementary school, feeding us, attending classes at graduate school, working a student job at the archive library, picking up my son, cooking dinner, and then getting back onto the couch. Weekends consisted of cooking, doing homework, and napping on the couch in between. I also read from the couch. I assisted with my son's homework from the couch. I entertained my son from the couch.

Every moment of the day was focused on when I could lay down on the couch, get back in bed, and steal a moment away to stare out the window. The couch became an inter-

WE WILL REST

vention accessible to me immediately. I didn't need to leave my home or travel from my city to retreat into a world outside the one I had already built. My body was my retreat. My site of liberation. My body is my home.

I enjoyed my physical home and the people in it, and the inexpensive couch that my husband bought when he got a small holiday bonus check from work. I woke up from a long nap in our actual bed one day after studying for two days straight for a final exam and he had snuck the new couch into our living room. The first time I saw it I knew it was special. After sitting down once on it, I immediately wanted to re-cline. So, I did. My refuge. It became a sacred object creating a powerful place of empowerment to connect with my Divine. My body attached to the couch became the deepest place of freedom as I demanded deliverance out of the bondage of grind culture.

Identify your sacred object. Do you have a couch? A favorite chair? A hammock? A yoga mat? A special blanket? A carpeted floor that becomes a massive rest space? Can you spend time on a porch sky gazing? Do you have an accessible outdoor area full of grass? I once napped every day on my lunch break at an oppressive call-center job in my car. But my couch! I craved it and it accepted me in all my tiredness and

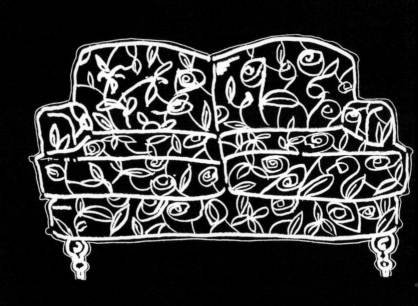

WE WILL REST

exhaustion. A ritual that lasted for months. This was the door and on the other side of it my escape artist life began. The portal that rest provides to those suffering under the weight of capitalism, white supremacy, and patriarchy. Rest wants us to see it as an escape, a refuge, and a guide. Unlearn the lies about what it means to labor in a culture so deeply unwell and sleep-deprived. Crawl if you must. Demand if you must. You must rest. ***The escape plan continues.***

In collaboration with my inexpensive couch was my bathtub. Shiny, slick white porcelain baptismal pool in a small bathroom. Vintage green tile on the floor and the lower half of the walls, a small window that was hard to pry open. I filled up the bathtub daily. Slowly pouring in potions and powders and hopes. Always ground oatmeal, lavender essential oil, Epsom salts, coconut oil, apple cider vinegar. Sometimes tears too. A small salty volume of tears blending and mixing slowly. Watching the hot water fill up was hypnotizing. Climbing in and feeling the water hug my skin was my baptism. This was when I reclaimed my body as my own. Reclaim your body. ***The escape plan continues.***

It's six a.m. and, as my eyes open wide, I realize I have slept through my alarm yet again. Most nights I went to bed in the "burning the midnight oil" hours. Falling asleep or, more accurately, passing out quickly as my eyelids got heavy while doing something else. I can count the times on one finger when the circumstances of my day allowed me to intentionally plan for bedtime. The robot mode of doing is so hard to deprogram from. It can feel like your entire world will crumble if you slow down even for a few hours. I connected my lack of money with how much laboring I could fit in one day even though I was overworking at two jobs sometimes. Poor people work more hours a week than most. The culture makes it almost impossible to believe you can thrive without internalizing capitalism.

I thought I would die. I thought the exhaustion of capitalism would crush me. Rest saved my life. Anyone in this culture who believes and feels they are enough right now has begun the escape artist transformation. A brave trickster and master teacher in faith and enough-ness in a culture that teaches us that there's never enough. A prophet. To know in the deepest parts of your soul that your birth grants you divinity, rest, care, and power is a seed planted in fertile ground. But you don't have to wait until you are fully knowing. You don't have to wait until you have found the light already inside you. It's there. You can come to rest and the path of escape by simply acknowledging that you are exhausted and it feels challenging to keep up with the unsustainable pace that capitalism demands. This awareness is also a seed in fertile ground.

The thing about me and other escape artists before me is this: I'm gonna thrive even when the world is on fire because my help doesn't come from this wicked world. Be a witness and rejoice in the representation of a Black woman who refuses to overwork, who says no constantly, and who doesn't view busyness as a badge of honor. I want to be a witness to your escape plans. My honor is centered in my humanity. I don't have to do anything else. There is life and rest outside of the constant need to grind and work constantly. Capitalism has a chokehold over our lives right now. The next second, the next minute, the next hour, is ours to refuse the grind. We can craft and build temporary spaces of joy and freedom here now.

Listen close: It's time to lay down. It will take deep subversion, dreaming, and community care. Can I hold your hand telepathically? May I lay you down on a bed made of love and orchids? Will you transform and prepare for escape with me? If you don't participate in the heavy lifting that grind culture demands and things fall apart because of this, let it fall. Trust your body. Trust Spirit. Trust community. Trust your Divine connection to power. Trust resurrection. Trust the infinite ways we can rest.

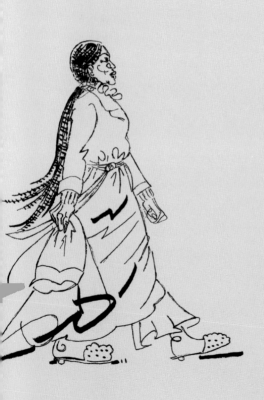

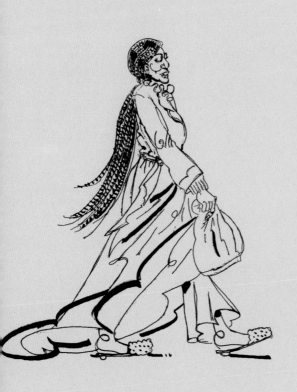

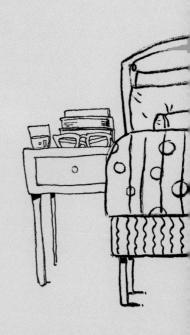

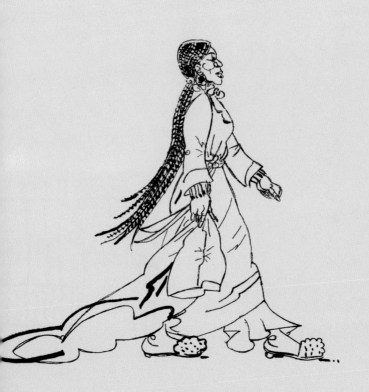

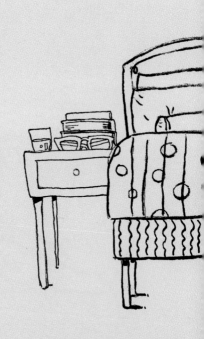

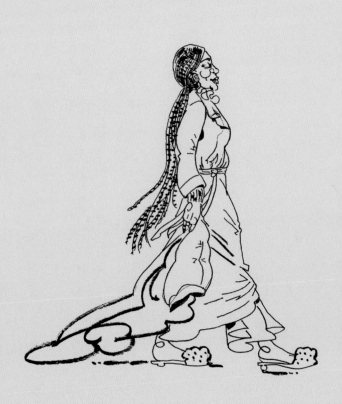

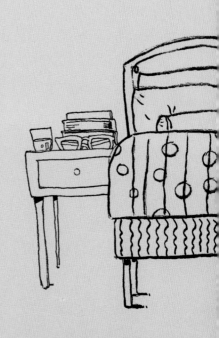

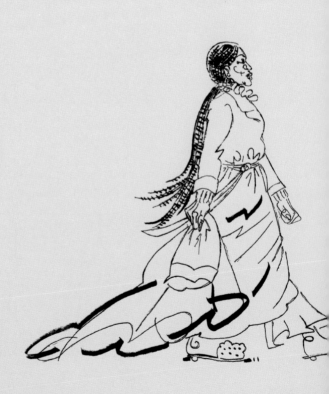

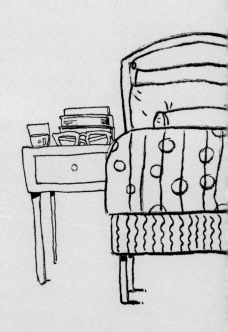

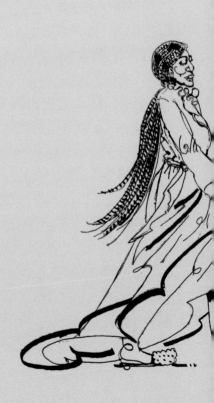

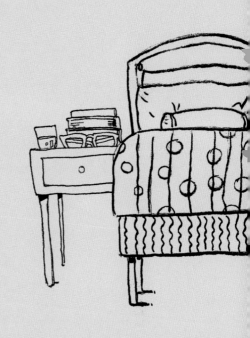

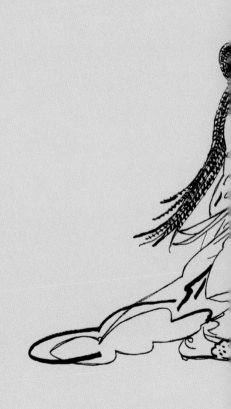

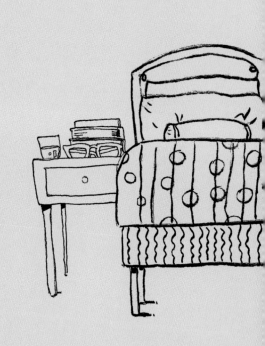

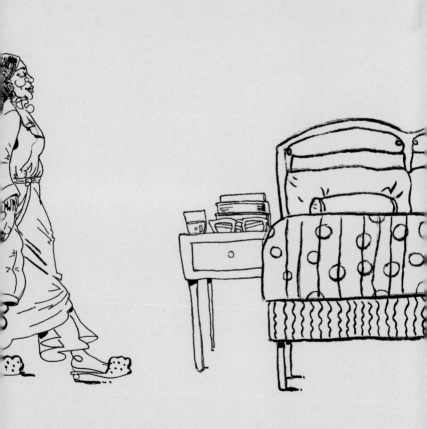

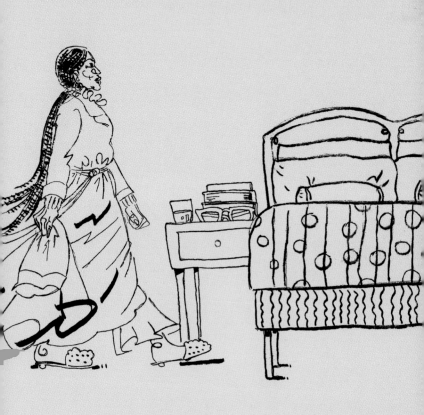

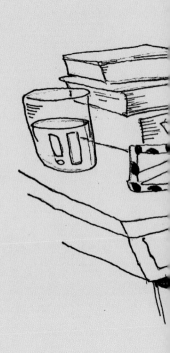

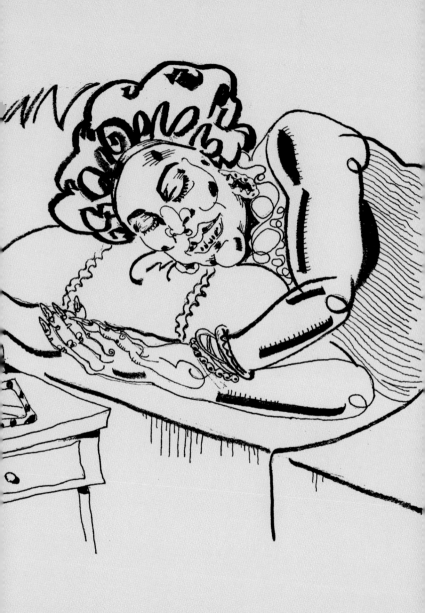

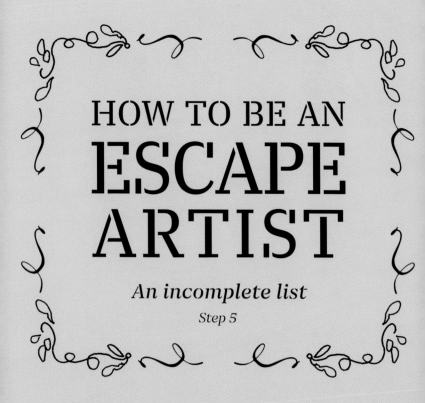

HOW TO BE AN ESCAPE ARTIST

An incomplete list

Step 5

WE WILL REST

Create a concise one-sentence response to the question "What are you willing to rest for?" Then memorize it. Embody it. Become it. Then lay down in the beauty and power of your plans.

Rest is a spiritual practice.

Rest is a justice practice.

Rest is a love practice.

Rest is a care practice.

Rest is a faith practice.

Rest is an anti-war practice.

Rest is an anti-capitalist practice.

Rest is a freedom-seeking practice.

Rest is a connection to the Creator.

Rest is a connection to your Ancestors.

Rest is a connection to Spirit.

Rest is a connection to Nature.

Rest is a connection to the Divine.

Rest is refusal.

Rest is life-giving.

Rest is power.

Rest is medicine.

Rest is heaven.

Rest is now.

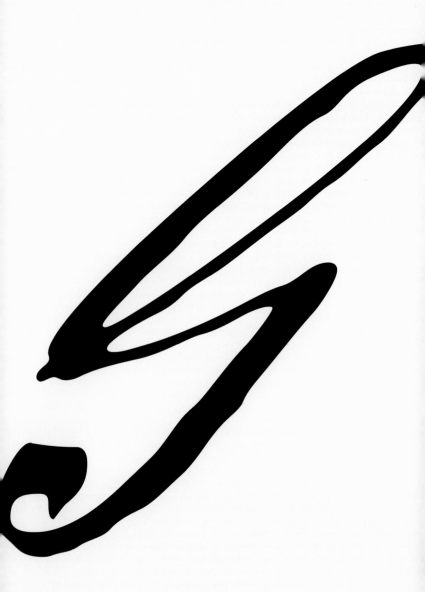

WE WILL REST

Grind culture has stolen our imagination. Our thinking is limited because we are deeply disconnected, exhausted, and sleep-deprived. We don't believe we are worthy of anything unless we burn ourselves out to accomplish it. Focus on the escape. Focus on the transformation. You can be free. You are free.

EVERYTH
IN F
AND E

G IS FAIR

EST

CAPE.

I got something to say
I got words that want to bounce around my mouth
I got secrets and truths and freedom things to scream
I got beautiful, smack-you-upside-your-head
words to throw

I want to cuddle
On a quilt of handmade paper
Shout the Holy Spirit out of my insides
With a tambourine
I will communicate with the Goddess of Rest
Then snatch her title for my own gratification

I licked a razor blade last night
My tongue begged for the attention
In the red of my room while my soul stared in jealousy
I watched words softly ease crawl over my body
Like an uninhibited freak-type lover

I no longer have any use for mere paper and pens
I want to tattoo poems on my forehead
Draw the alphabet with black eyeliner inside my thighs
On my breasts
I will scribble haikus in blood

I want rest to speak for me

My tongue is healing from the razor-blade incident

I am twelve months pregnant with silence

I want to give birth

Name my seed RESTED POTENTIAL

I tied my arms behind my back this morning

Forced myself to memorize my own voice

I digitally recorded my dreams

Made a mixtape full of leisure

I'm selling it on trains and buses

I got things I need to get off my chest

I am sick of shame riding my back

I only have enough strength

To carry my heavy tongue

I only have enough power to rest

Hold on

Hold on to your faith

Hold on to your tenderness

Hold on to your hopes

Hold on to rest

Hold on

Hold on

Hold on

Hold on to this book

Hold on to your dancing

Hold on to your body

Hold on to your neighbor

Hold on to the heaven inside

In a culture like ours, built on grinding and capitalism, it is a scary proposition to slow down. In your slowing down, you will only gain a sense of peace, justice, and liberation. To reclaim time.

It is scary. It is hard. It is alchemy. Our lives are beautiful resistance. We survived birth, bombs, and blood.

Creator, help us know this daily. Help us lean into our brilliance and magic. Teach us how to be an escape artist. Rewind us back to our beginnings. The moment that was just rest. Unleash the Divine power into our life. Make us a vessel. Give us strength. Give us rest. Give us softness. Give us confidence. The systems should be rejoicing that we are alive, whole and Divine. We don't owe these made-up violent systems anything. Be in service to yourself first. Be you. Escaping is worth it.

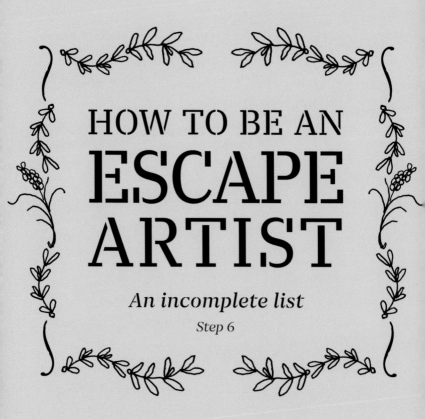

HOW TO BE AN ESCAPE ARTIST

An incomplete list

Step 6

Listen. You must slow down to listen. Listen to your body. Listen to your heart. Listen to the birds. Listen to the wind. Listen to your dreams. Listen for clues. Your escape from grind culture depends on listening.

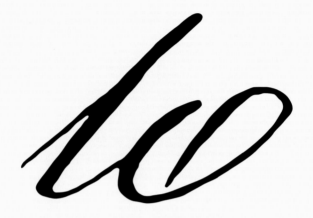

We Will Rest! Our mantra. Our call. Our protest song. A justice manual. Devotional. Liberation text. Resistance material. Sing it from the rooftops. Sing it like you mean it. Make it a lullaby. Dream it. A daily dose of love. Tuck it away in your heart. Dream it. Dream so effortlessly that you become human again. Your machine-like ways are burned in a heap of rubble, and we warm ourselves from the flames. This is the way forward. Machine-like programming no more. A rested world is a healed world. I want to dream possibilities forever.

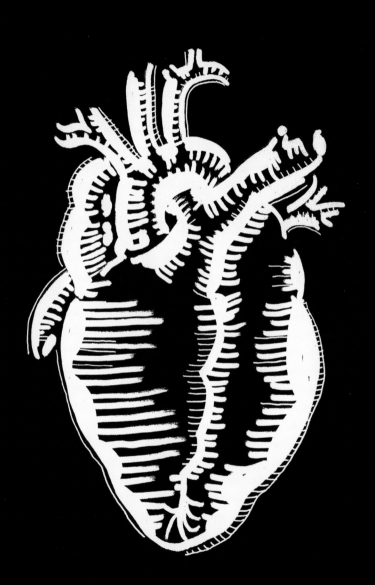

TRICIA HERSEY

Let this be

A MEDITATION
ABOUT RESURRECTION

Let this be

A MEDITATION
ABOUT REDEMPTION

Let it be

A MEDITATION
ABOUT RESTORATION

Let it be

A RE-IMAGINATION

WE WILL REST

I come from a lineage of Black women who:

Poured holy oil in shoes and on foreheads

Wrapped salty bacon on wounds

Made pots of beans and rice to feed a multitude

Buried dead babies while praising God

Rattled tambourines in pews

Altar called their lost husbands back to Creator

Believed in the healing of your body

by laying hands

Rebuked the devil with tongues

Knew you were pregnant before you did

Called the Holy Spirt "the ghost" as a pet name

Turned off all electricity while it was storming

Thankful to be an apprentice

Grateful for this part of my DNA

May I always remember who I am

May I always rest

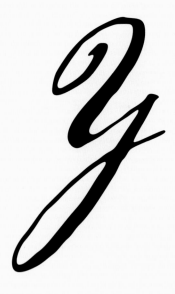

You believe it is normal and necessary to have trauma residing in your body because capitalism placed it there. The body was not built to burn out. What we call burnout is trauma.

WE WILL REST

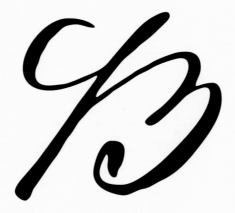

Burnout is a scam and its language was created by agents of grind culture, guided by corporations tricking you into believing it's a normal and regular part of any working person's career. We speak the word "burnout" so much when it should be named correctly instead. There is no "burnout." There is worker exploitation, abuse from capitalism, and trauma stored in our bodies from a lifetime of overworking.

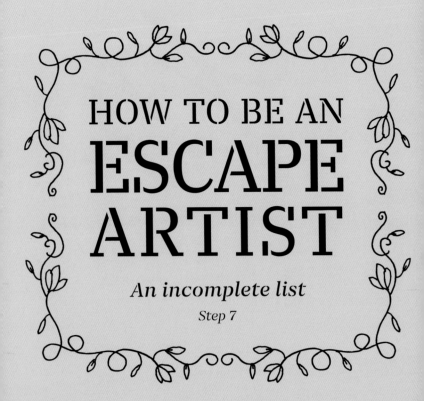

HOW TO BE AN ESCAPE ARTIST

An incomplete list

Step 7

WE WILL REST

Reinvent yourself over and over again. Resurrect yourself over and over again. Focus daily on the spectacle of escape. The best spectacles are the ones that are organic and catch everyone off guard. Don't be afraid to say less. Every word doesn't have to be used. Silence is holy and goes directly to the point. Silence is rest. People need to know that you are pissed about the bamboozlement. Let grind culture know you are not playing around. This is not a game or a time to shrink. Your thriving depends on the art of escape.

AN ESCAPE PRACTICE

Every day, morning or night, or whenever you can steal away, find silence. Even if for only a few minutes. Look for quiet time, quiet breathing, quiet wind, quiet air. It is there. Even if it's cultivated in your body by syncing with your own heart beating. Guilt and shame will be a formidable and likely opponent in your resistance. We expect guilt and shame to surface. Let them come. We rest through it. We commit to our subversive stunts of silence, truth, daydreaming, community care, naps, sleep, play, leisure, boundaries, and space. Be passionate about escape.

Make us new!

The dead now walk.

It's night no more.

And rest comes in the morning.

There is a space between waiting

and redemption.

A breathing room.

Be not afraid of the dark.

Let the rage become soft petals dropping

onto your forehead.

A warm bed awaits.

May you forever rest peacefully there.

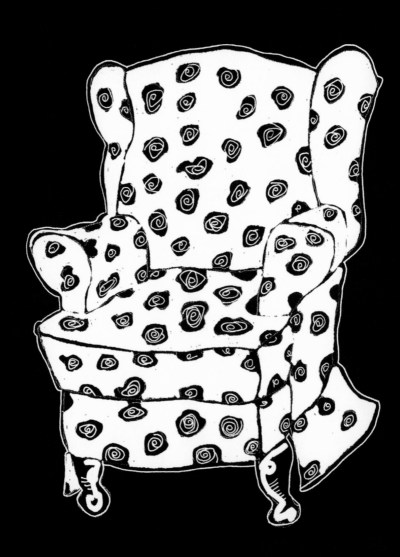

WE WILL REST

This is the story of an exhausted, curious Black woman who one day decided to build a world outside the one forced on her. Her world includes a soft space to rest. A cocoon away from the world that doesn't see who she truly is. A wicked world viewing her body the way it regards a cranking metal machine: no bones, no heart, no skin, no brain. But she has strong fragile bones, an open beating heart, warm skin, and a brain blessed by downloads from above. She has wings that can fly because my Ancestors blow air to power wings. Her wings spread with the energy of hummingbird wings. This is the story of a Black woman traumatized from capitalism, white supremacy, and patriarchy, so she decided to never be held hostage by the beast of grind culture again. This is the story of an escape artist, a young trickster, a survivalist who decided that resting is the only goal.

I
AM
FROM

WE WILL REST

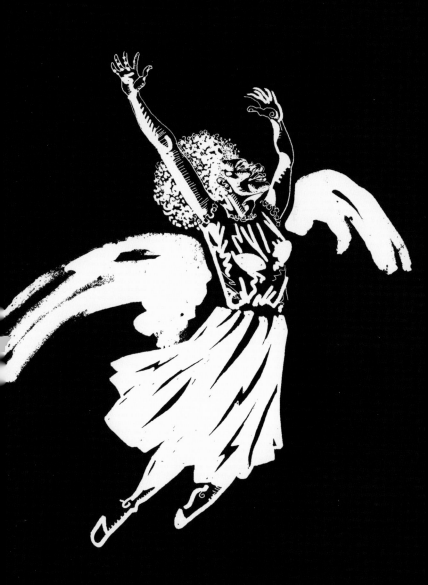

I am from the continent of Africa

Afro Alien without a confirmed country

I feel Ghana in my bones tho

By way of Mississippi and Louisiana

By way of Chicago

City of big bloody shoulders

Sharecroppers way deep in rural southern lands

Body bent breaking bleeding bright

Great Migration stories wrap us like a vintage quilt

Gospel music blaring on a clock radio

In my mother's small yellow kitchen

From trauma remixed to resistance

Resistance turned into power

Power now my freedom

Rest now my liberation

I escape

I am from the inside of every liberation text

My skin a living archive resting

I am from Pentecostal tent revivals

My daddy's booming voice preaching

Fish fries and BBQ dinners

Mama napping every day in a La-Z-Boy recliner

From steel mill–working father and uncles

Ready to reimagine what we can do with our bodies

They belong to us, correct?

From high school sweetheart mama and daddy

Who have never cursed a bad word

Sweet, tender brown beings floating around and over my head

I am from holy dreams

Large wishes folded up

In pockets and purses

I am the hope

On the other side

The beautiful resistance side

I am from Great-Grandma Rhodie's apron

Pistol tucked to protect her eighteen children from demonic eyes

I come from the portal of rest

Holding me up

Laying me down

Liberation my middle name

Rest the prototype

Rest my resurrection

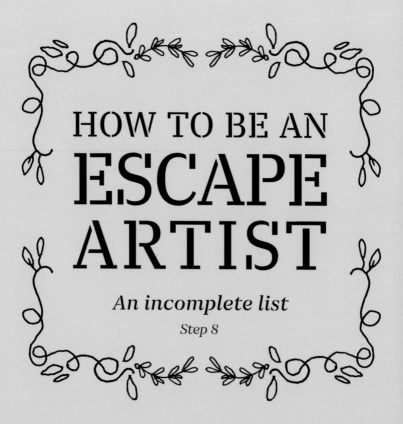

HOW TO BE AN ESCAPE ARTIST

An incomplete list

Step 8

Start being okay with being seen as an outsider to grind culture. An outlier wizard. Embrace the mystery. Why would you want to be a part of exhaustion, disembodiment, and trauma? Why would you want to align with and trust in toxic capitalism and consumerism as both sell self-care as expensive things and doing more? Don't be fooled. Rest your eyes right now. Take a nap right now. Daydream right now. Sky gaze right now. Make being on the outside a freedom space. Hide in plain sight.

I am live and direct from the cracks of late-stage
capitalism.

I escaped the lies. I escaped the terror.

From the wind of my Ancestors blowing me into a
DreamSpace, I float on.

We are here from the Planet of Hope! The Planet
of Rest!

Thank you, Divine Being!

TO BE AN OUTLIER
TO GRIND CULTURE
REQUIRES
FLEXIBILITY,
GRACE,
AND A TRICKSTER
ENERGY.

ODE TO MY FAVORITE ESCAPE ARTIST
HENRY BOX BROWN

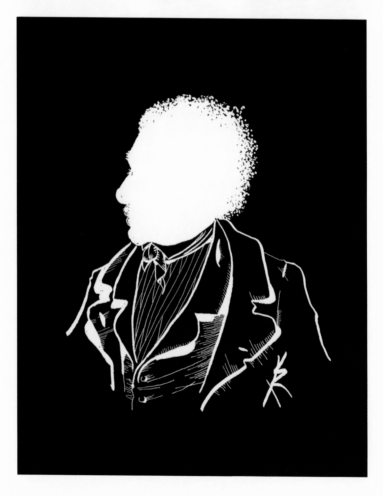

WE WILL REST

This is the story of Henry Box Brown. The ultimate escape artist. My inspiration. Maybe he will inspire you too. He had a plan. He had a vision. He had his body. My obsession with the concept of escape came when I was a young girl in the fourth grade. A lesson during Black History Month was on Henry Box Brown. Mrs. Young began, "Today, class, we will be learning about a man named Henry Box Brown. He mailed himself to freedom in a box."

On March 23, 1849, a man named Henry Box Brown was nailed into a large wooden postal crate marked "this side up with care" and mailed from slavery in Richmond, VA, to freedom in Philadelphia, a voyage of two hundred and fifty miles. Twenty-six hours later, he emerged from this box singing a psalm of thanksgiving, and he would never again be a slave.

—*The Many Resurrections of Henry Box Brown*

by MARTHA J. CUTTER

I hold on to the blueprint of Henry as a plotting magician, hope lecturer, liberation wizard, performance artist, and escape artist. For my next trick, I will pull a freeman out of a box. For our next trick, we will disrupt grind culture by creating sacred spaces to rest and slow down. I will never be a slave to grind culture. I will never ignore the pleas from my body and Spirit to slow down. Henry emerging from the hiding place of a three-foot-long and two-foot-six-inch-deep box singing a song of thanksgiving. Breathing the pure air of freedom. Rejoicing in the light of Philadelphia. Trusting and loving his body for bending, stretching, and being bold in collaboration with him. His site of liberation as he held his head down, rested his back against the box shifting as he traveled an entire day plus some on trains. At two hundred pounds and five feet eight inches, the journey stuffed inside a box nearly killed him. The same way grind culture is slowly killing us. The way the pace of my life nearly killed me.

Ode to the tricksters. Ode to the ones ready to leap and to those on the edge barefoot with their toes clutching. A red carpet will not be rolled out with an invitation for us to rest from our toxic, hustle-focused culture. Sit with that. Lay with this. Take all the time you need to accept this sad truth. Grieve forever. Then rejoice in your plotting and in your plans. Rejoice in your escape making by closing your eyes. You can rest. Nothing is impossible. Come back to your center. Move your limbs. Open your chest. Think about the infinite power we have as individuals and communities. The holy happens there. Go there.

Henry Box Brown told very few about his escape plans. A few humans along the railroad journey and a few at his final stop in Philadelphia cultivated the ultimate practice of community care. Who would ever believe this possible? Who would ever believe that a body and mind could withstand this. But who would believe that we withstand overworking, sleep deprivation, and the trauma of capitalism daily as we ignore and push ourselves? You will have to prepare to love yourself and to refuse to inflict violence onto yourself by overworking. You can pop out of your own metaphorical box singing a song of redemption and gratefulness. You can bend rest into a heart-shaped light. Attach it to a tank top with safety pins. Let love glow through us like running water. Let rest scribble a map in the sand to guide us to our escape.

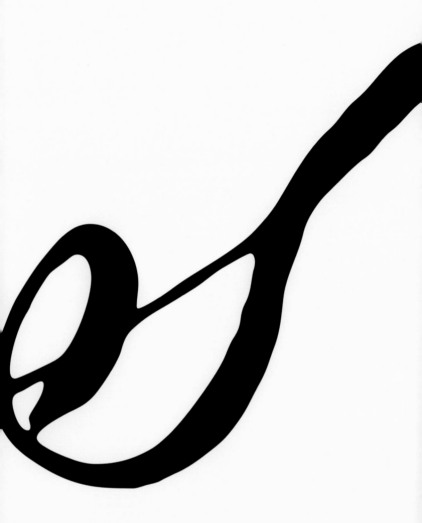

WE WILL REST

Say this aloud: "My body is a brilliant, beautiful, inventive, high-technology vessel of power and liberation granting me the energy and space to just be." We can just be. We are beautiful. We are enough. We are Divine. We have time. We have time to rest. We Will Rest!

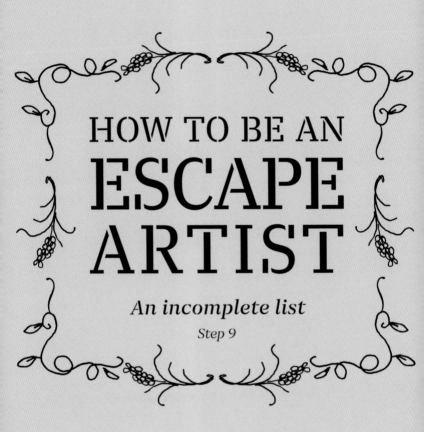

HOW TO BE AN ESCAPE ARTIST

An incomplete list

Step 9

WE WILL REST

Read a poem daily. You will need it for your dreaming mission and your escape maps. May I recommend Lucille Clifton, Nikki Giovanni, Langston Hughes, or Audre Lorde? Write your own. A prompt to start: "My rest feels like…"

Your devotional

Your daily dose of resistance

Material for you to dream with

Your star in the skies

Carry it in your bag

Hide it in your dressers

Sing it as a song from the rooftops

Sing it like you mean it

Make it a lullaby

Dream rest

Dream delicately

Easily become human again

Shed your machine-like ways

We will rest

We will escape

Vulnerable soft prayers.

Weep now. Grieve now.

Water the pages.

Water your exhausted heart.

Rest.

To grieve is to be alive.

To escape you must grieve.

THE RUINS

Sometimes life boils over

Like rice cooked on a stove too fast

Like a pot of collards simmering

You put in too much water

The top shakes

Rattles

Stove is now ruined

I'm into ruining things

I will ruin all plans created without my consent

about what my body can withstand

I will ruin the image of the mule and savior to all

Maybe destruction is the first real step toward

building new

Toward getting things to make sense

Even the people who you think are free ain't free

Straddling the line, making their plans up as they go

In the ring and showing up

Capitalism can't ruin me anymore

May sleep cradle and soothe the righteous tonight.

May we follow the light in the stars.

May we follow the light within.

May our dreams reveal everything we need.

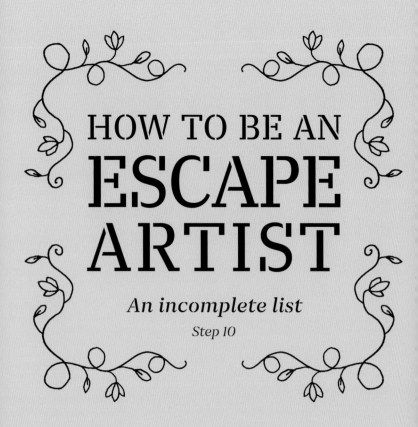

HOW TO BE AN ESCAPE ARTIST

An incomplete list

Step 10

WE WILL REST

Create an escape map. Keep creating them for the rest of your days. Trace the path telepathically. Write the plans down on scraps of paper, then tuck and hide them away. Find them by surprise. When you need the map, it will appear. Create a map for the following: How to bend time, How to sky gaze, How to daydream, How to rest.

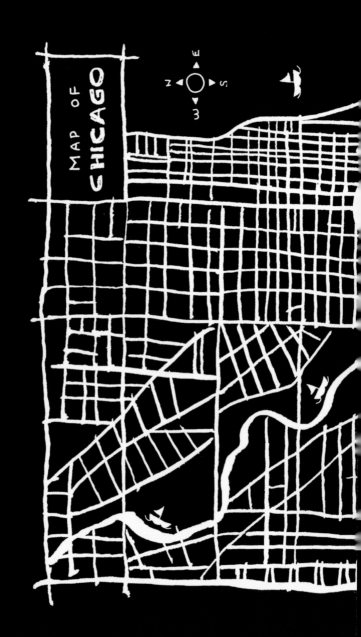

MAP OF **CHICAGO**

N E S W

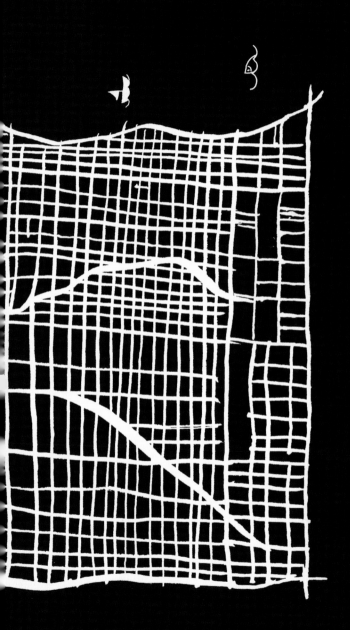

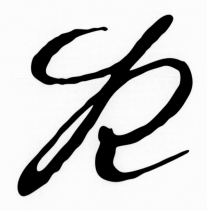

Rest is a prayer.

Rest is a holy place.

WE WILL REST

The road to hell is paved
with good intentions.
May my path be lit
with burning Divine love.
May I create my heaven right
here on Earth in a fluffy bed.
May the mirror be my blueprint.
May my Ancestors drive me to liberation.
May I gather up all the exhausted souls
under a white floating tent.

Fly us away.
Fly us to a rested planet.
May care be right here beside us.
May we hold each other's lavender-soaked hands.
May we place our burdens
on the altar of rest.
Float away.
Float away.

DO YOU R
WHAT IT
TO W
AND DA

WE WILL REST

MEMBER
ELS LIKE
NDER
REAM?

Stop holding on to the lies that you've been taught. Stop holding on to anything that gets in the way of thriving. The thing you are so fearful of losing may be your blessing in disguise. Let that burn. Build anew. Rest. Let go of people pleasing. Let go of overextending. Let go of guilt. Let go of shame. Be like Henry! Prepare to lose disconnection. Prepare to be an escape artist.

This is the way to softness in a hard world. I remember moments when I was a young girl. My memory like a camera. There are so many moments from the time I was eight until high school involving my imagination. I was always imagining another world, always singing, and always creating. One day I sat in the grass of an abandoned lot on my block. The kids in the neighborhood turned this space overgrown with weeds into a way to shorten our walks home from school. I would cut through the tall grass, but one day I decided to sit down. Then the sitting turned into resting flat on my back as the summer wind blew over me. I gazed at the blue sky and white clouds. I watched them pass by and felt hypnotized. A butterfly fluttered overhead and as it landed on a weed next to me, I stared at every detail. The little brown pieces of the body, the softness of the wings, and its small size. The way it bounced without a care in the world.

Oh, how the sun and the air felt so different. It felt like I could see things hidden. I remember the chirping of the birds and how comforting and calm it felt. I always seem to remember childhood things like the smell of my mama's coffee in the morning, the smells of her cooking for Daddy, the times I just wandered around without a schedule, not on a timeline, not rushing, and not thinking about what I had to do. I would simply be open to what the day would bring. The moments before the brainwashing took root in my Spirit and body. We need mental clarity. We need pleasure and joy. We need rest. We need to escape.

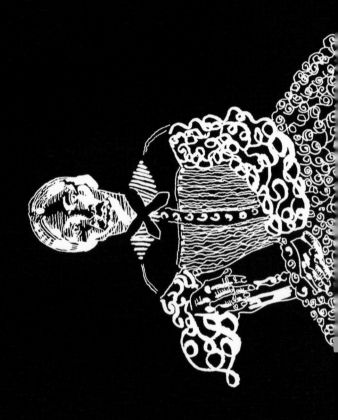

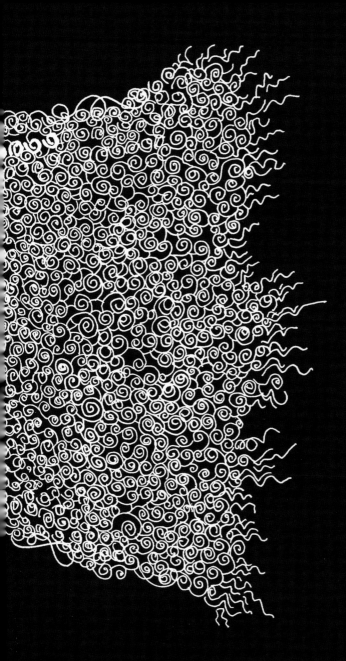

HALL of FAME
of ESCAPE ARTISTS

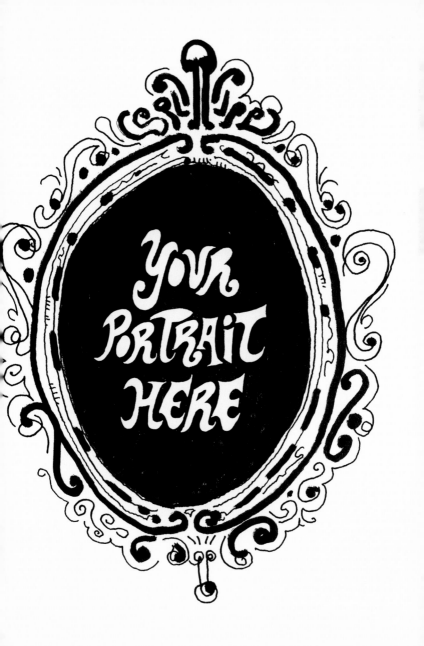

The book you are holding is an artifact.

Flee!

An escape plan is before you.

An escape plan is written in ink.

On your heart.

On these pages.

On your DNA.

Everything is soft here.

Everything is held by others here.

There are hands linking hearts.

Breathing syncing.

Everything is easy here.

Everything is soft here.

Rest is the way to softness in a hard world.

ABOUT
THE AUTHOR

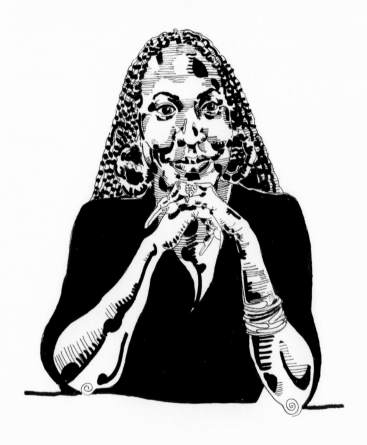

WE WILL REST

Tricia Hersey is a multidisciplinary artist, theologian, escape artist and founder of The Nap Ministry. She is the global pioneer and originator of the "rest as resistance" and "rest as reparations" frameworks, and collaborates with communities all over the world to create sacred spaces where the liberatory, restorative, and disruptive power of rest can take hold. Tricia's work is seeded within the soils of Black radical thought, somatics, Afrofuturism, womanism, and liberation theology. She is a Chicago native who believes in daydreaming, porch sitting, and poetry.

Tricia's work is deeply influenced by her experiences as the daughter of an abolitionist pastor, as a native of the South Side of Chicago, and as the torch-bearer of her family's Mississippi and Louisiana roots. She necessarily dissolves these boundaries to unlock mental, physical, and spiritual spaces for radical thought and imagination. The wideness of her practice opens portals and possibilities of world-building and future-casting.

Tricia's words and the immersive experiences she creates through and outside of The Nap Ministry are calling us to move far beyond mainstream concepts of wellness. She asks us to study the ways in which our divinity, higher purpose, and ability to resist violent and oppressive systems are intertwined with how we access our rest, imagination, and DreamSpace. Her work is a pathway to the rest practices needed to collectively build and imagine new worlds as we simultaneously dismantle and deprogram ourselves from the systems that prop up and perpetuate the racial, social, and environmental harm done by white supremacy and extractive capitalism.